Homœopathy is a system of medicine which recognises our uniqueness. We are all individuals with particular strengths and weaknesses, so it isn't surprising that when we become ill we each react in our own way. Even if we catch the "same" cold as our neighbour or colleague, our response to it may be quite different from theirs.

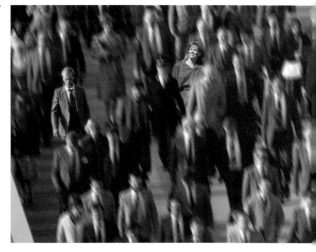

Using the time-honoured principle that like can be cured with like, homœopathy has taken a wide range of natural substances and carefully recorded the symptoms these substances cause in healthy people. Matching these substances, as closely as possible, to the individual and the particular symptoms that they are experiencing encourages their own healing energy to return them to health. The results are often remarkable, bringing about cures that are rapid, gentle and permanent.

What is homœopathy?

Although it was first described by Hippocrates 2,500 years ago, homœopathy as it is practised today evolved 200 years ago. The word comes from the Greek and means similar suffering. This refers to the central philosophy that a substance that can produce symptoms in a healthy person, can cure those symptoms in a sick person. For example, a person suffering from hayfever might be given a remedy prepared from an onion, because a healthy person chopping an onion usually experiences watering eyes and irritation. Similarly, someone suffering from insomnia might be given a homœopathic dose of coffee.

Is homœopathy safe?

Yes. Since the substances are given in minute doses unwanted side-effects are avoided, making them safe to use even in situations where conventional drugs would be dangerous or inadvisable, for example during pregnancy or when treating infants.

How does it work?

Although there is a great deal of empirical evidence that homœopathy does work, nobody yet knows how. Those who are sceptical point out that homœopathic remedies are often so dilute that not even a molecule of the original substance remains and so conclude that any beneficial response is probably due to the placebo effect. This explanation seems unlikely as experiments have shown homœopathic medicines to be equally effective in the treatment of animals.

The answer to this mystery is likely to be found by those studying quantum physics and electro-magnetism. The production of homœopathic medicines involves two processes: dilution and succussion (shaking and striking against a surface). It is thought likely that these combined processes leave an imprint of the original substance's energy pattern in the dilutant. This energy imprint, given in homœopathic medicine, somehow stimulates the body's own healing energy to start working.

How does homœopathy differ from conventional medicine?

Homœopathy is an holistic medicine. This means that its focus is on the whole person. Spiritual, mental, emotional and physical factors are regarded as completely inter-connected and no single factor is taken in isolation. It is based on the idea that symptoms are not the cause of disease, they merely show that "dis-ease" exists. Symptoms are the body's way of warning us that all is not well and are attempting to restore balance.

A simple analogy is to imagine that you are driving your car and the red oil warning-light comes on. You know nothing about cars so you decide to take it to the garage. When you come to pick up the car, the light is no longer on, so, having paid the bill, you drive off quite happily. You naturally assume the problem is fixed, but would you feel so satisfied if you later discovered that the garage had merely unscrewed the warning-light bulb?

Homœopathy is a truly holistic medicine because it uses symptoms as helpful indicators which can be used as guides to treating the individual and their "dis-ease". Instead of merely removing the symptoms, it removes the central disturbance in the individual's energetic balance. Once this has been done the symptoms disappear anyway, because the warnings they were trying to give have become unnecessary.

Can I take homœopathic medicine if I'm already taking other medication?

Yes, it is perfectly safe to do so. However, you should not attempt to reduce your other medication without supervision from a qualified homœopath or doctor.
See page 26.

What kind of things can I treat myself?

As you will see from this booklet, with very little effort, the home-prescriber can treat a wide variety of injuries or acute illnesses. To qualify as "acute" an illness should develop quickly and have three phases. At first, you just don't feel quite right; then there are strong recognisable symptoms; followed later by the convalescent stage where the symptoms begin to improve. Examples of acute illnesses are coughs; colds; conjunctivitis; cystitis; flu; gastric flu; food poisoning; measles; mumps; chickenpox; travel sickness etc.

Why should I have a broad selection of remedies at home.

Injuries and acute illnesses, by their very nature, happen at unpredictable times when it may be difficult or impossible to buy what you need. It is therefore a very good idea to have a complete range of medicines 'on standby'. The more you have the easier it will be to make the best match between the symptoms and the remedy that can cure them. If you are going away remember to pack them.

When should I consult a qualified homœopath?

If you have a serious or recurring condition or you have had a number of acute illnesses recently, it is always best to see a qualified homœopath. Remember homœopathy can be used to treat anything, even problems that have no clear diagnosis, because it treats the individual rather than the disease. For information on finding a qualified homœopath and a description of how they work, see page 24.

BEFORE YOU BEGIN TO PRESCRIBE:

THERE ARE **TWO IMPORTANT LAWS** THAT YOU NEED TO FOLLOW TO USE HOMŒOPATHIC MEDICINES SUCCESSFULLY:

THE LAW OF SIMILARS means matching the symptom picture of an illness or injury to the symptom picture of the medicine. To help you do just that, this booklet has two distinct sections. Complaints you can treat are described first, followed by a Mini Materia Medica. This describes, briefly, the symptom pictures of 36 frequently-needed remedies. Begin by looking up the complaint you want to treat and noting which remedies may help. Next, before prescribing, turn to the Mini Materia Medica and see which description most closely fits the person you are treating. If you have given two or three doses of a particular remedy without any reaction, it was probably the wrong choice. It won't have done any harm, but you should try to find a remedy that matches the over-all picture better.

THE LAW OF THE MINIMUM DOSE means using as little of a medicine as possible to stimulate the body's own healing mechanism. Give one dose (in this case one small pill) and wait to see what relief it brings. If you have a reaction to the remedy (either an improvement or an aggravation of symptoms) do not take any more medicine. Only repeat the dose if the symptoms stop improving before a full recovery is reached or if the same symptoms return (i.e. the case relapses). If the symptoms change significantly select a new remedy to fit the new picture. If in any doubt, **wait**. Giving the body more medicine than it needs will not improve or speed up the action of the medicine, if anything it may stop the medicine from being effective.

By using these two laws homœopathy provides a completely individual prescription and dosage that treats each person's "dis-ease" as unique to them.

OTHER FACTORS TO CONSIDER:

ANTIDOTING

Certain substances are known to antidote certain homœopathic medicines in some people. It is therefore advisable to avoid these substances if possible: Coffee (including decaffeinated), mint (notably in toothpaste), camphor, menthol, eucalyptus (often found in vapour rubs and cold remedies). Keep remedies in a cool dark place away from strong odours (and small children).

TAKING THE MEDICINES

Homœopathic medicines are delicate and need careful handling. Touch them as little as possible. Shake one pill into the lid of the bottle and put it directly under the tongue of the person taking the medicine. If possible the dose should be taken fifteen minutes before or after having anything to eat or drink, cleaning your teeth or smoking. Obviously this does not apply in an emergency where it should be taken as soon as possible. You can crush and dissolve remedies in water and sip them, but do not swallow the pill down with water, tea or coffee. Before repeating the dose, please consider the Law of the Minimum Dose (opposite) carefully. If symptoms show no improvement or return persistently always consult a qualified homœopath. Homœopaths have more than 1,000 remedies at their disposal and can treat the underlying weakness in the individual's constitution.

If you already see a homœopath regularly, please discuss self-prescribing with them.

SAFETY FIRST

Serious injuries and illnesses should never be treated without seeking expert advice. Use your instincts and common sense, if you are worried call for help first, then give the appropriate remedy whilst you are waiting for help to arrive. If in any doubt check for these...

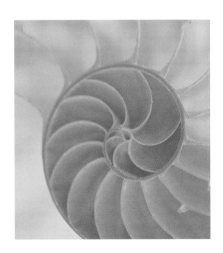

WARNING SIGNS

If the person you are treating has any of the following seek assistance immediately:

backache, or fever, with urinary infection

bleeding, heavy or unexplained

breathing, rapid shallow or difficult

burns, severe or larger than your hand

chest pain, severe

confusion, following trauma or over-exposure to sun

consciousness, lost or impaired

convulsions

delirium

dehydration, especially in babies, small children and elderly

drowsiness, unexplained or unexpected

headache, severe

fever, above 103.5F / 40C or persistent or with stiff neck

fits

fluid, watery / bloody, from ears or nose following head injury

movement, full range, lost or impaired

puncture wounds, near vital organs

speech, lost or impaired

stool, pale or white

streaks, red running away from a wound

swelling, rapid or severe (especially of mouth or throat)

thirstlessness, prolonged with fever or diarrhoea or vomiting

urine, profuse or scanty or bloody

vision, lost or impaired

vomiting, unexpected and repeated

wheezing, severe

yellowness, of skin or eyes

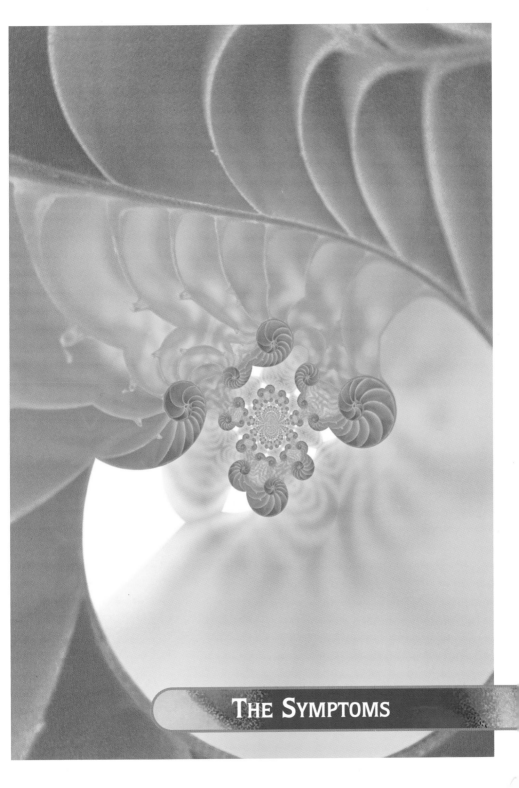

THE SYMPTOMS

SOME COMMON COMPLAINTS YOU CAN TREAT

Please remember, to prescribe accurately and effectively it is important to read the description of the remedy in the Mini Materia Medica that follows this section, before making your selection.

ACCIDENTS

(see BROKEN BONES, FRACTURES, INJURIES & WOUNDS)

Give immediately, **Arnica 30c.** Where there is shock or swelling alternate **Arnica 30c** with any other indicated remedies, repeating as often as necessary.

ANXIETY

With fever, **Aconite 30c** or **Arsenicum 30c.**
Anticipatory, with diarrhoea, **Gelsemium 30c.**
With paralysis or trembling, **Gelsemium 30c.**

see also:
Anticipatory, with diarrhoea, **Arg Nit 30c.**
Anticipatory, **Lycopodium 30c.**

ASSAULTS

For fear, **Aconite 30c.**

For shock, **Arnica 30c**.

BITES & STINGS

(see SEPSIS)
Red, hot, swollen, better cold applications, **Apis 30c.**
Animal bites, with shooting nerve pain, **Hypericum 30c.**
Blue, cold, puffy, better cold applications, **Ledum 30c.**

see also:
Bluish around bite, **Lachesis 30c.**
Very painful, worse touch, **Staphisagria 30c.**

BLOOD BLISTERS

After injury **Arnica 30c**

BOILS

Small, numerous and sore, **Arnica 30c.**
Burning, **Arsenicum 30c.** Hot and throbbing, **Belladonna 30c.** Slow to heal, **Silica 30c.**

see also:
Itchy, **Sulphur 30c.** Painful, infected, with pus, **Hepar Sulph 30c.** If symptoms persist consult a qualified homœopath or doctor.

BREAST FEEDING DIFFICULTIES

Hard, engorged, hot, red, **Belladonna 30c.**
Hard, engorged, hot, pale, worse movement, **Bryonia 30c.** Abscess with smelly, corrosive pus, **Merc Viv 30c.** Too much milk, **Pulsatilla 30c.**
Sharp pains in left breast during feeding, **Silica 30c.**
Abscess which is very slow to heal, **Silica 30c.**

Baby vomits / has colic after breast milk, **Silica 30c.**
see also:
If abscess with pus, extremely painful, **Hepar Sulph 30c.**
also recommended:
If milk production varies greatly, **Urtica Urens 30c.**
If sore, cracked nipples, radiating pains, **Phytolacca 30c.** If too little milk, **Dulcamara 30c.**

BROKEN BONES

(see FRACTURES)
Before setting, **Arnica 30c.**
Worse for slightest movement, stitching pains, **Bryonia 30c.**

also recommended:
Only after setting, both **Symphytum 6c**, one dose nightly & **Calc Phos 6x**, one dose mornings for 7 days.

BRUISES

Of soft tissue, **Arnica 30c.** (see also Arnica cream)
also recommended:

Arnica cream / ointment, but only on unbroken skin. For deep tissue (e.g. contusion of breasts), **Bellis Perennis 30c.**

BURNS

For shock, **Arnica 30c.**
If area of injury better cold applications, **Cantharis 30c.**
If area of injury better hot applications, **Arsenicum 30c.**

see also:
For deep burns, which are slow to heal, **Kali Bich 30c.**
also recommended:
Urtica Urens cream externally to soothe minor burns.
For serious burns, seek medical assistance immediately.

CHICKENPOX

Feverish and fearful, **Aconite 30c.**
With fever and throbbing head, **Belladonna 30c.**
If blisters pus-filled / smelly, **Merc viv 30c.**
With cough, thirstless, clingy, **Pulsatilla 30c.**
Very itchy rash, extreme restlessness, **Rhus tox 30c.**

see also:
Rash slow to emerge, with cough, **Ant tart 30c.**
also recommended:
Use **Calendula Cream / Ointment** or Talc externally, but wait until rash emerges fully.

CHILLBLAINS

Hot, itchy, worse heat, **Pulsatilla 30c.**
Dark red inflammation, worse cold, damp, **Rhus Tox 30c.**

also recommended:
Worse on the feet, worse for cold, **Agaricus 30c;**
Tamus cream / ointment externally
Calendula cream/ointment externally, if they break.

COLDS

Early stages, **Aconite 30c.** Thin, watery, burning discharge, chilliness, **Arsenicum 30c.** With flu-like aching, thirstless, **Gelsemium 30c.** Thick, bland, profuse discharge, thirstless, **Pulsatilla 30c.**

Slow to go, **Silica 30c.**
see also:
Thick, yellow, stringy discharge, **Kali Bich 30c.**
With sneezing and dripping nose, **Natrum Mur 30c.**

COLD SORES

On lips, **Rhus Tox 30c.**

see also:
On lips, mouth, caused by sun, **Natrum Mur 30c.**
On lips, **Sepia 30c.**

COLIC

Better bending forwards, **Belladonna 30c.**
With fever and cramps, **Nux Vom 30c.**
Better lying still with knees up, **Bryonia 30c.**

see also:
For pain relief, **Mag Phos 30c.** If complaint comes on after humiliation, **Staphisagria 30c.**

CONSTIPATION

Great dryness / thirst, sometimes with headache, **Bryonia 30c.** With ineffectual urging, unfinished sensation, **Nux Vom 30c.** During pregnancy, **Nux Vom 30c.** With "shy" stool that slips back, **Silica 30c.**

see also:
Hard, knotty stool, **Lycopodium 30c.** Stools like sheep dung (small balls), **Natrum Mur 30c.**
If sensation of a lump, not better after stool, **Sepia 30c.**
Large dry stool, with painful straining, **Sulphur 30c.**

COUGHS

After exposure to dry, cold wind, **Aconite 30c.**
Dry cough with chest pain and headache, **Bryonia 30c.**
Dry at night, loose in the morning, **Pulsatilla 30c.**
see also:
Loud, rattling, (whooping) cough with vomiting,

Ant Tart 30c. With blue face, vomiting mucus, **Drosera 30C.** With nosebleeds, **Drosera 30c** or **Ipecac 30c.** With hoarse / sore throat, **Hepar Sulph 30c.** With blueness, stiffness, nausea, vomiting, **Ipecac 30c.** With ropy, sticky expectoration in the morning, **Kali Bich 30c.**

CROUP

First choice, reduces accompanying fear, **Aconite 30c.**
see also:
Attacks in the early hours, **Hepar Sulph 30c.**

On waking, with lump sensation, **Lachesis 30c.**
also recommended:
If Aconite fails, attack is around midnight, **Spongia 30c.**

CUTS

(see WOUNDS)

CYSTITIS

Burning when urinating, **Apis 30c.**
Cutting / burning before, during or after urination, **Cantharis 30c.** Burning during / after urination, worse if lying, **Pulsatilla 30c.**

see also:
After sexual intercourse, **Staphisagria 30c.**
If symptoms persist consult a qualified homœopath or doctor.

DENTAL TREATMENT

Before if fearful, **Aconite 30c.**
Before fillings or extractions, **Arnica 30c.**
Bleeding gums, after, **Arnica 30c.**
To treat after effects of, **Arnica 30c.**

Shooting nerve pain after, **Hypericum 30c.** Flu or cold symptoms after mercury fillings, **Merc Viv 30c.**
see also:
For sore, cut gums, **Calendula 30c** or **Staphisagria 30c.**

DIARRHOEA

With vomiting, caused by food poisoning, **Arsenicum 30c.** Like chopped spinach, with teething, **Chamomilla 30c.** With anticipatory anxiety, **Gelsemium 30c.**

see also:
With anticipatory anxiety, **Arg Nit 30c.** For exhaustion after, **China 30c.** Only on waking, **Sulphur 30c.**

EARACHE

From cold, severe pain, restlessness, fear, **Aconite 30c.** Stinging pain, worse swallowing, **Apis 30c.** Throbbing pain, with high temperature, **Belladonna 30c.** Unbearable pain, worse windy weather, **Chamomilla 30c.** After swimming, **Chamomilla 30c.** With smelly blood-streaked discharge, **Merc Viv 30c.** Itching inside ear, increased swallowing, **Nux Vom 30c.** Ear red externally, **Pulsatilla 30c.** After measles, **Pulsatilla 30c.**

see also:
Throbbing pain in slow teethers, **Calc Carb 30c.** Stitching pain, smelly discharge, **Hepar Sulph 30c.** Stitching pain, worse left, **Kali Bich 30c.** With sore throat, worse left side, **Lachesis 30c.** Spasmodic, shooting pain, **Mag Phos 30c.** If blocked with hard wax, **Silica 30c.** With painful noises in the ear, **Sulphur 30c.**

EXAMINATION NERVES

(see ANXIETY)
With diarrhoea / trembling / paralysis, **Gelsemium 30c.**

see also:
With diarrhoea / hurried feeling, **Arg Nit 30c,** better once exams.

EXHAUSTION

Following physical over-exertion, **Arnica 30c**.
see also:

If after dehydration, **China 30c**.
also recommended:
If nervous exhaustion, **Kali Phos 6x**.

EYE INFLAMMATION

Upper and lower lids red and puffy, tears hot, **Apis 30c**. Thick, yellow smelly discharge, with a cold, **Pulsatilla 30c**. With watering, caused by a blocked tear duct, **Silica 30c**.

see also:
Eyes red, smelly yellow discharge, **Arg Nit 30c**.
also recommended:
Bathe in diluted tincture of **Euphrasia or Hypercal**.

EYE INJURIES

(see EYE INFLAMMATION)
Fear after, **Aconite 30c**. bruising and / or shock, **Arnica 30c**. Black eye, **Ledum 30c**.

also recommended:
If Arnica fails and injury is to eyeball itself, **Symphytum 30c**. If with feelings of anger, **Staphisagria 30c**.

EYE STRAIN

With weak vision, pains aching or burning, **Ruta 30c**.

FOOD POISONING

Particularly after meat, **Arsenicum 30c**. After bad fish, **Pulsatilla 30c**.

see also:
If after shellfish, **Lycopodium 30c**.

FLU

(see COMMON COLD & GASTRIC FLU)
Burning fever with chills, restless, **Arsenicum 30c**.
Feverish and irritable, lies very still, **Bryonia 30c**.
Total physical prostration with shivering,
Gelsemium 30c. Pains in bones, joints, chilliness,
Nux Vom 30c. Aching, with restlessness, red-

tipped tongue, **Rhus Tox 30c**.
see also:
Pains in bones, back, legs, **Ipecac 30c**.
also recommended:
Bone pains, great thirst, **Eupatorium Per 30c**.

FRACTURES

(see BROKEN BONES)
If pain and swelling are severe, **Arnica 30c**.

With shooting nerve pains, **Hypericum 30c**.
If slightest movement causes severe pain, **Bryonia 30c**.

GASTRIC FLU

(see COMMON COLD & FLU)
Restless, feverish and / or chilled, diarrhoea,
Arsenicum 30c. Mouth tastes bitter, **Bryonia 30c**.
With chilliness and irritability, **Nux Vom 30c**.

see also:
Constant nausea, not better for vomiting, **Ipecac 30c**.
also recommended:
With thirst before vomiting, **Eupatorium Per 30c**.

HAEMORRHOIDS

Caused by pregnancy, **Nux Vom 30c**.
also recommended:
If large, bleeding, **Hamamelis 30c**.

If large, **Kali Carb 30c**.
With burning, especially after stool, **Nit Ac 30c**.

HANGOVERS

Caused by cigarette smoke, **Ignatia 30c.**
Indigestion after too much beer, **Kali Bich 30c.**

With sick headache and /or nausea, **Nux Vom 30c.**

HEADACHE

From getting chilled, **Aconite 30c.** From shock / fright, **Aconite 30c.** With sudden, violent onset, **Aconite 30c** or **Belladonna 30c.** After over-excitement or exertion, **Arsenicum 30c.** After washing hair, **Belladonna 30c.** Throbbing headache during period, **Belladonna 30c.** Throbbing headache from too much sun, **Belladonna 30c.** After change in the weather, **Bryonia 30c.** With dry cough, **Bryonia 30c.** With slow onset, **Bryonia 30c** or **Gelsemium 30c.** With violent pain at the back of the head, **Gelsemium 30c.** Due to grief, **Ignatia 30c.** Sensation as if a nail were driven into head, **Ignatia 30c.** In small spots, caused by sinusitus, **Kali Bich 30c.** With a cold, **Merc Viv 30c** or **Nux Vom 30c.** After too much rich food or alcohol, **Nux Vom 30c.** After loss of sleep, **Nux Vom 30c.** After eating ice-cream, **Pulsatilla 30c.** After change in the weather, especially to damp, **Rhus Tox 30c.** After getting wet, **Rhus Tox 30c.** From working in artificial light, **Silica 30c.** From draughts, **Silica 30c.** From travelling, **Silica 30c.**

see also:
If before a thunderstorm, **Phosphorus 30c.** With hunger before or during, **Phosphorus 30c.** Due to grief, **Natrum Mur 30c.** After eye-strain, **Lycopodium 30c** or **Natrum Mur 30c.** From working in artificial light, **Sepia 30c.**

also recommended:
If due to disturbed sleep patterns, **Cocculus 30c.**
If symptoms persist consult a qualified homœopath or doctor.

HEAD INJURIES

Give immediately, **Arnica 30c.**
also recommended:
If never been well since, **Natrum Sulph 30c.**

If symptoms persist consult a qualified homœopath or doctor.
(see WARNING SIGNS)

HIVES

With fever, **Apis 30c.**

With burning, itching, stinging, **Rhus Tox 30c.**

INJURIES TO

Head, **Arnica 30c. (see HEAD INJURIES)**
Muscles, **Arnica 30c. (see also SPRAINS)**
Soft tissue, **Arnica 30c.** Coccyx, **Hypericum 30c.**
Spine, **Hypericum 30c.** Nerve-rich areas (e.g fingers / toes), **Hypericum 30c.** Bones, **Ruta 30c.**

(see also broken bones / fractures)
Palms of hands, **Ledum 30c.** Soles of feet, **Ledum 30c.** Tendons / ligaments, **Rhus Tox 30c** or **Ruta 30c.** Shins or bones near surface, **Ruta 30c.**
also recommended:
For breasts / deep tissue, **Bellis Per 30c.**

INJURIES WITH

Fear, **Aconite 30c.** Long-lasting after-effects, **Arnica 30c.**

Shock, **Arnica 30c.** Splinters, **Silica 30c.**

INOCULATIONS

Before, reduces local reaction, **Hypericum 30c, Ledum 30c.** To treat the puncture wound, **Ledum 30c.** Shooting pains after, **Hypericum 30c.**
Any other reactions consult a qualified homœopath or doctor.

JET-LAG

For exhaustion, **Arnica 30c.**
With sense of paralysis, **Gelsemium 30c.**

also recommended:
For disturbed sleep patterns, **Cocculus 30c.**

MEASLES

(see EYE INFLAMMATION)
Sudden on-set with burning, itchy rash, **Aconite 30c.** With eye inflammation, **Apis 30c** or **Pulsatilla 30c.** Bright red rash with hot dry skin, **Belladonna 30c.** Slow onset, with headache or dry cough, **Bryonia 30c.** Face dark red, back of head aches, drowsy, **Gelsemium 30c.** Earache after measles, **Pulsatilla 30c.**.

see also:
With purulent discharge from eyes and / or ears, **Kali Bich 30c.** Purple rash, slow to emerge, **Sulphur 30c.**

also recommended:
Burning tears, photophobia, **Euphrasia 30c.** or bathe in diluted tincture.

MENSTRUAL PROBLEMS

Late / scanty after a fright or becoming chilled, **Aconite 30c.** Hot, heavy blood loss, **Belladonna 30c.** Period late after getting feet wet, **Pulsatilla 30c.** Nausea and faintness with period pains, **Nux Vom 30c.**

see also:
Constant nausea before and during period, **Ipecac 30c.** Pains worse before period starts, **Lachesis 30c.** Cramping pains, **Mag Phos 30c.** Headaches before / during period, **Natrum Mur 30c.** Bearing down pains, **Sepia 30c.**

MOUTH ULCERS

Caused by burn from hot food, **Cantharis 30c.** Painful, increased saliva, offensive breath, **Merc Viv. 30c.**

also recommended:
If on the tongue, **Nit Ac 30c.**

MUMPS

With fever, restlessness and anxiety, **Aconite 30c.** With high fever, painful hot parotids, **Belladonna 30c.** Hard, enlarged glands, worse on right, **Merc Viv 30c.** If breasts, ovaries or testicles are affected, **Pulsatilla 30c.** Swollen parotids, worse on left, **Rhus Tox 30c.**

Better for heat, worse for cold, **Silica 30c.**
see also:
If breasts, ovaries or testicles are affected, **Carbo Veg 30c.** Face red and swollen, worse left, **Lachesis 30c.**, Moving from right to left, **Lycopodium 30c.**

NOSEBLEEDS

After shock or injury, **Arnica 30c.**

see also:
With cough, **Ipecac 30c.**

LABOUR PAINS

With fear that she will die in childbirth, **Aconite 30c.** Intolerable, infuriating, **Chamomilla 30c.** Weak, with back pain, **Gelsemium 30c.** Ineffective, with weepiness, "Help me", **Pulsatilla 30c.**

also recommended:
Most homœopathic pharmacies will supply you with a childbirth kit full of useful remedies for before, during and after labour.

POST-NATAL CARE

OF BABY: If baby is breast-fed mother may take the remedy, if not hold pill inside baby's lower lip until it takes effect.
Shock, after fast violent birth, **Aconite 30c.** Retention of urine, **Aconite 30c.** Blocked tear duct, **Silica 30c.**
see also:
In cases of apparent asphyxia, **Ant tart 30c.** or **Carbo veg 30c.**

also recommended:
In cases of apparent asphyxia, **Laurocerasus 30c.** OF MOTHER: In all cases, for exhaustion / after-effects, **Arnica 30c.** repeated. Disturbed sleep / after-effects of medication, **Chamomilla 30c.** Shooting pains from damage to perineum, **Hypericum 30c.** After injuries to coccyx, **Hypericum 30c.**

Continued overleaf

see also:

For cuts, tears or grazes, **Calendula 30c** or bathe in tincture. Exhaustion after severe blood loss, **China 30c.** Bright red, hot, profuse bleeding, **Ipecac 30c.** Bright red flow of blood, **Phosphorus 30c.**

After Caesareans, **(see SURGICAL OPERATIONS)** After episiotomies, **Staphisagria 30c.**

also recommended:

After forceps deliveries / Caesareans, **Bellis Per 30c.** After any deep / internal bruising, **Bellis Per 30c.**

Scalds

(see BURNS)

Better for cold applications, **Cantharis 30c.**

Sepsis

If red, hot, throbbing, (to stop sepsis), **Belladonna 30c.** With blood-streaked, corrosive pus, **Merc Viv 30c.** When slow to heal, **Silica 30c.**

see also:

Painful with pus, to drain in early stages, **Hepar Sulph 30c.**

Shock

With fearfulness, **Aconite 30c.** Following trauma, accidents etc, **Arnica 30c.**

From receiving (bad) news, **Gelsemium 30c.** Emotional, **Ignatia 30c.**

Sore Throats

Dry, red, burning, **Aconite 30c.** Burning, stinging pains with great swelling, **Apis 30c.** Dry, red, hot with (painful) desire to swallow, **Belladonna 30c.** Shooting pains to right ear on swallowing, **Belladonna 30c.** With swollen glands, **Belladonna 30c** or **Silica 30c.** Dry throat and mouth, with thirst, **Bryonia 30c.** Slow onset, flu-like aching and weakness, **Gelsemium 30c.** With increased salivation and bad breath, **Merc Viv 30c.** With hair sensation on back of tongue, **Silica 30c.**

see also:

With lost voice due to overuse, **Arg Nit 30c.** Sensation of fish-bone / splinter / crumb, **Hepar Sulph 30c.** Ulcerated tonsils with stringy discharge, **Kali Bich 30c.** Pain worse swallowing saliva than solids, **Lachesis 30c.** Left side first (may move to right), **Lachesis 30c.** Right side first (may move to left), **Lycopodium 30c.**

also recommended:

Tonsils swollen, worse for hot drinks, **Phytolacca 30c.**

Sinus Problems

Inflammation of frontal sinuses, **Merc Viv 30c.** Blocked up sensation, worse in a warm room, **Pulsatilla 30c.** Nose dry, blocked and sore, **Silica 30c.**

see also:

Pain in spots, sticky yellow-green mucus, **Kali Bich 30c.** With headache, worse on right side, **Lycopodium 30c.**

Splinters

To ease them out, **Silica 30c.**

Sprains & Strains

To reduce swelling, **Arnica 30c.** If worse for slightest movement, **Bryonia 30c.**

Worse first, yet better continued movement, **Rhus Tox 30c.** Worse lying on affected part, **Ruta 30c.**

Stiff Neck

Caused by draughts, lifting, **Rhus Tox 30.** **see also:** If caused by lifting, **Calc Carb 30c.**

If symptoms persist or there is high temperature consult a qualified homœopath or doctor

STOMACHACHE

(see COLIC)

STYES

(see EYE INFLAMMATION)
Eye is red, the lid is painful and swollen, **Apis 30c.**
Eye itch, lids sticky, yellow-green discharge,

Pulsatilla 30c.
If pus is present, (see SEPSIS)

SUNBURN

Skin is dry, hot, red, throbbing, painful, **Belladonna 30c.** If severe, take as soon as possible, **Cantharis 30c.**

SUNSTROKE

With fever and / or headache, **Belladonna 30c.**
If symptoms much worse for movement, **Bryonia 30c.**

also recommended:
With faintness and headache better for pressure,
Glonoin 30c.

SURGICAL OPERATIONS

In preparation for, **Arnica 30c.** To counter the
after-effects of, **Arnica 30c.** For surgical wounds
with nerve pain, **Hypericum 30c.** After
amputations, **Hypericum 30c.**
see also:
For surgical wounds, **Calendula 30c** or

Staphisagria 30c.
After catheters, enemas, **Staphisagria 30c.**
For bad reaction to anaesthetic, **Phosphorus 30c.**
For painful trapped wind after surgery, **China 30c.**
also recommended:
If deep tissue is affected, **Bellis Per 30c.**

TEETHING PROBLEMS

Red, hot cheeks, with restlessness, **Aconite 30c.** Red,
hot swollen cheeks, **Belladonna 30c.** Red, hot cheek
or cheeks, bad-tempered, **Chamomilla 30c.** With
green stool, **Chamomilla 30c.** Better cold drinks, fresh

air, **Pulsatilla 30c.** If teething is slow, **Silica 30c.**
see also:
If teething is slow or delayed, **Calc Carb 30c.**
If better external heat, **Mag Phos 30c.**

TRAVEL SICKNESS

Better for vomiting, but finds it difficult, **Nux Vom 30c.**
also recommended:

Worse for fresh air, better lying down, **Cocculus 30c.**
With heavy head, worse for fresh air, **Petroleum 30c.**
Better for fresh air, **Tabacum 30c.**

VACCINATIONS

(see INOCULATIONS)

VOMITING

With diarrhoea, **Arsenicum 30c.** Caused by over-
indulgence, **Nux Vom 30c.** In breast or bottle-fed
babies, **Silica 30c.**
see also:
With retching cough, **Ant Tart 30c** (see COUGHS).

After, for exhaustion caused by dehydration, **China 30c.**
With cough, vomiting mucus, **Drosera 30c** (see
COUGHS). Worse for coughing, **Ipecac 30c** (see
COUGHS). With constant nausea, not relieved by
vomiting, **Ipecac 30c.** If approximately 15 minutes
after cold drink, **Phosphorus 30c.**

WHIPLASH

With shooting nerve pain, **Hypericum 30c.** Deep ligament / tendon injuries, possible tearing, **Ruta 30c.**

WOUNDS

Cuts, grazes, sores, **Calendula 30c.** Incised, clean
cuts, **Hypericum 30c.** Lacerations, **Hypericum 30c.**

see also:
For surgical wounds, **Staphisagria 30c.**

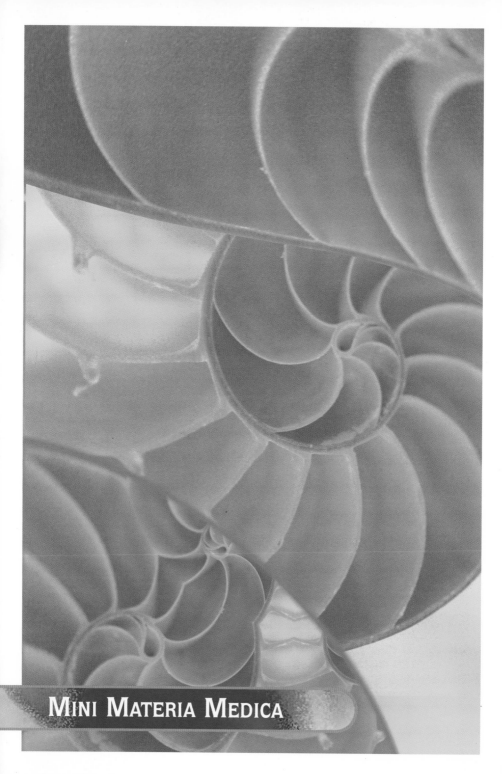

MINI MATERIA MEDICA

Please note: No. 1 Remedy = Most frequently prescribed. To ensure your prescribing is as accurate as possible always match the symptoms as closely as possible to the medicine.

ACONITE

No. 1 Remedy for nipping colds in the bud. Useful in the early stages of colds, fevers, inflammations. Suits healthy people whose complaints come on suddenly. Possible causes: cold / dry wind ; fright / shock. Characterised by extreme restlessness and fear. May specifically have an unfounded fear of death. Dry, hot skin. Symptoms worse evening / around midnight. Thirsty for cold drinks. May say everything tastes bitter, except water. Better: fresh air. Worse: touch.

APIS

No. 1 Remedy for bites and stings. For the remedy to be effective symptoms should generally fit the following picture: Oedematous swellings. Redness. Pains burning and stinging. Restlessness. Thirstlessness. Better: cold applications. Worse: heat; 4-6pm.

ANT TART

Important (rattling) cough remedy, where patient is unable to expectorate (cf. Ipecac) and is "drowning in mucus". Feels suffocated, weak, drowsy and limp. May be irritable. Much yawning and sweating. Tongue is coated white. Better: expectoration; sitting up; cold drinks. Worse: warmth; lying down; 4pm; company

ARG NIT

No. 1 Remedy for fear of flying. Useful for anticipatory anxiety and gastro-intestinal problems (belching / flatulence). Suits warm-blooded people with a tendency to feel hurried and impulsive. They may have a fear of failure when having to perform in public. Their fear is justified, as they often rush through things and get into a mess. (cf Gelsemium & Lycopodium). Pains splinter-like. Better: open air; walking fast. Worse: crowds; sweets (gets diarrhoea).

ARNICA

No. 1 Remedy for accidents / shock / physical exhaustion. Should be a first choice after most accidents, injuries or physical ordeals. Given early it will reduce swelling and bruising. Patient has a fear of being touched, because of the pain and may want to be left alone. May claim to be alright when they clearly are not. Classic response of someone in shock. Upper body is hot, whilst lower is cold. Memory may also be poor. Better: lying down, with head low. Worse: jarring; lying on injured part.

ARSENICUM

No. 1 Remedy for food poisoning. Characterised by great physical prostration with mental restlessness. Patient does not want to be left alone. May have a fear of death. Pains and discharges are burning, yet the patient feels chilly and all symptoms, except headache, are better for heat. Thirsty for frequent sips of usually hot drinks. Better: warmth; lying down. Worse: midnight - 3am.

BELLADONNA

No.1 Remedy for very high fevers. Inflamed area or entire patient (!) is burning, red and hot. The eyes are glassy and the pupils dilated. Onset of complaints is sudden. Possible cause: chill to the head. Pains are violent and throbbing. Rapid pulse. Patient is angry, may be delirious and even have visions. Thirsty, may crave lemonade. Better: lying down. Worse: touch or jarring movement; 3pm.

Bryonia

No. 1 Remedy for dry, painful coughs.
Dryness of all mucous membranes. Great thirst for large amounts at long intervals (opposite of Arsenicum). Patient lies absolutely still; all symptoms are much worse for the slightest movement. Pains are stitching. A "bear with a sore head" who is irritable and resentful of being questioned or fussed over. Better: firm pressure. Worse: 9pm; after eating cabbage or beans.

Calc Carb

No. 1 Remedy for slow, difficult teething.
Often needed when growing up or going through major developmental changes. Classically fat, fair and flabby. Chilly. Easily over-exerted and very sweaty (esp. back of head). Sour-smelling. May fear many things (e.g. the dark; monsters; animals; insects). Slow developers, particularly poor at assimilating their food, which may cause problems in bone and teeth formation. Crave boiled eggs. Better: constipation; dry weather. Worse: heights; getting cold or wet; teething; milk.

Calendula

No. 1 Remedy for healing wounds.
Very useful first-aid remedy for cuts; superficial burns or scalds; ulcers; scalp wounds; after teeth extraction or childbirth. It stimulates formation of healthy scar tissue (without lumps). Use externally in cream, ointment or tincture form. Take internally if there is much discomfort or suppuration (cf. Hepar Sulph). Better: warmth; walking or lying absolutely still. Worse: damp dull weather; evening.

Cantharis

No. 1 Remedy for the intense pain of burns.
Often effective in the treatment of cystitis, where there are burning pains before, during and after urination. Intense mental and physical irritation. Onset is sudden and violent. Pains are cutting and burning. Patients have a burning, intense thirst, but are worse after drinking (especially cold drinks). Better: cold applications. Worse: touch.

Carbo Veg

No. 1 Remedy for resuscitation.
"The homœopathic corpse reviver". This remedy has saved many lives. Symptoms at their most extreme are complete state of collapse due to oxygen starvation. Body (even breath) is cold. May appear limp, pale or blue. Less severe cases have extreme sluggishness. Many digestive disorders, especially wind. (cf. Lycopodium) Upper abdomen / stomach very bloated. May be brought on by over-indulgence. Better: cool air; being fanned; burping. Worse: warmth; dehydration; before sleep; tight clothing.

Chamomilla

No. 1 Remedy for teething children.
Especially if child has one red cheek. Characterised by over-sensitivity. Pains are intolerable and appear to be out of all proportion to the illness or injury. Suited to bad-tempered children who are only quiet when carried and constantly request, then reject things. They are hot and sweaty (especially the head). Better: for being uncovered. Worse: 9pm - midnight.

China

No. 1 Remedy for de-hydration.
Delicate types whose senses are too acute. Emotionally and physically exhausted. Complaints often arise after loss of fluids / severe dehydration (e.g. after fever or diarrhoea). Bloated abdomen, but not relieved by burping (cf. Carbo veg). Better: hard pressure; lying down; fasting; loose clothes. Worse: light touch.

Drosera

No.1 Remedy for whooping cough.
Excellent (whooping) cough remedy (see also Ant tart & Ipecac), where cough is violent, spasmodic and leads to gagging / vomiting or nosebleed (cf. Ipecac). Better holding chest. Sensation of feather in throat. Restlessness. Emotionally stubborn or suspicious. All symptoms improve after midnight. Better: sitting up; open air. Worse: lying down; talking; warmth.

GELSEMIUM

No. 1 Remedy for flu.
Especially if there is shivering up and down the spine. Characterised by paralysis. The remedy is known as the "glass coffin" because although there is complete physical prostration, it is coupled with mental alertness. Patient trembles, has aching muscles and heaviness especially of the head and eyes - even the eyelids droop. Better: for sweating or urination. Worse: physical exertion.

HEPAR SULPH

No. 1 Remedy for painful, infected wounds.
Characterised by hyper-sensitivity to everything: pain; touch; cold; noise; exertion. One of the chilliest known remedies. Emotionally can be violent and intense. Tendency to form pus. Pains stitching and splinter-like (cf Arg Nit). Better: heat; damp; lying in warm bed. Worse: uncovering; cold.

HYPERICUM

No. 1 Remedy for injury to nerves.
Useful first aid treatment for lacerated wounds from sharp instruments or any injury to nerve-rich areas (e.g. slamming door on fingers or falling on the coccyx). Pains are extreme and shoot along the nerves. Reputed anti-tetanus properties. Worse: motion or pressure.

IGNATIA

No. 1 Remedy for recent bereavement / emotional shock. Useful for treating symptoms which follow acute loss, grief or disappointed love. May not be able to accept what has happened and reacts with a sense of disbelief. Other signs may include hiccoughs, involuntary sighing or yawning. Can be used to treat fainting and hysteria. Better: warmth. Worse: tobacco; fresh air.

IPECAC

No. 1 Remedy for constant, violent nausea.
Vomiting brings no relief. Sudden bright red haemorrhages (nosebleeds; piles; periods). Spasmodic respiratory complaints. Dry cough with choking / gagging, difficulty expectorating (cf Ant Tart). Thirstless. Constant salivation and clean tongue. Better: open air. Worse: over-eating.

KALI BICH

No. 1 Remedy for painful sinuses.
Excellent remedy for colds and sinusitis, although chronic sinusitis is best treated by a qualified homœopath. Its main characteristic is a very stringy, sticky thick yellow / green discharge, which smells (cf. Pulsatilla). Suits those who become ill after getting chilled and are chilly whilst sick. Despite this chilliness they feel worse in summer. Pains are often in a small well-defined spot, but they can "wander". Better: warmth. Worse: on waking; at night; after eating.

LACHESIS

Left-sided complaints or begin on left, move to right (especially sore throats). Warm-blooded. Talkative, amusing but with an over-active mind. Can be suspicious and jealous. Intense. Better: open air; cold drinks; during or after period. Worse: menopause; alcohol; anything tight around the neck; after sleep; heat; heavy weather.

LEDUM

No. 1 Remedy for puncture wounds and black eyes.
Like Hypericum has reputed anti-tetanus properties. Use to treat deep wounds (e.g. those caused by nails) and bites from both animals and insects. Pains are sticking, tearing and throbbing. Area is swollen, blue and cold but, strangely, feels hot to the sufferer. Better: cold applications. Worse: heat.

LYCOPODIUM

Anxious. Lack self confidence especially when doing new things / speaking in public. Fine once they get started (cf. Arg Nit who hurries too much and does fail). Can be charming, but may be dictatorial at home. Complaints right-sided or move from right to left (opposite of Lachesis). Lots of wind. Bloated stomach and abdomen. Tendency to flatulence. Better: warm drinks; sweets; motion; open air; passing wind. Worse 4pm-8pm.

MAG PHOS

Known as **the homœopathic aspirin**. Very effective if crushed in warm water and sipped. Useful for neuralgia of the head and face, cramping or shooting pains. Relieves headaches; toothaches; menstrual pain. Those who respond well to this remedy may be sensitive or nervous types who often talk about their pains. Always seek professional homœopathic treatment if symptoms persist. Better: heat; firm pressure. Worse: cold; uncovering; touch.

MERC VIV

No. 1 Remedy for mouth ulcers.
Suits those people who are human thermometers, incredibly sensitive to both heat and cold and better moderate temperatures. They have very smelly breath and discharges (which may be streaked with blood). They are prone to swollen glands / colds and sweat profusely. Excessive saliva, especially at night, but they are extremely thirsty. Worse: in bed at night.

NATRUM MUR

No. 1 Remedy for cold sores.
If on the lips (with no other strong symptoms). Very sensitive people who remember the smallest slights for a long time. Feel everything so acutely they tend to protect themselves by shutting themselves off. They feel worse for consolation, except from a chosen few (or one). An important remedy for silent grief (the stiff upper lip). The middle of the lower lip may be deeply cracked. Discharges like egg white. Crave salt. Better: lying down; resting; sweating. Worse: heat, especially of the sun.

NUX VOMICA

No. 1 Remedy for hang-overs
... and over-indulgence in rich food. People who need this remedy are very chilly. Emotionally they tend to be tense, irritable and over-sensitive. They suffer from digestive complaints and although they feel much better for vomiting, they find it difficult to do so. They often work and play very hard, surviving on a "diet" of coffee, alcohol and tobacco, despite the effect it has on them. For best results take the remedy a few hours before going to bed. Better: rest; warmth and hot drinks. Worse: in the morning.

PHOSPHORUS

Lovely, bubbly, affectionate and sympathetic types. Unfortunately their poor boundaries mean they can become exhausted by the problems of others. Overly impressionable. Riddled with fears and anxiety. Burning heat and pains. Tendency to bleed easily. Desire spicy food; ice-cream. Better: cold drinks; eating; sleep (even a short nap). Worse: sudden weather change (especially storms); missing a meal; lying on left side.

PULSATILLA

No. 1 Remedy for childhood ear infections.
With this remedy the symptoms and the patients themselves are very changeable. Emotionally they are moody, tearful and crave company. Children are clingy and whine. Pulsatilla types are thirstless and are much worse for being in a stuffy room; their mood improves dramatically when they go out in the fresh air. Discharges are thick, bland and yellow-green. Complaints may come on after getting wet, chilled feet. Better: bathing; crying; movement; pressure. Worse: twilight; wet, windy weather.

SEPIA

Useful remedy for conditions brought about by hormonal changes in women. Suits those who are worn out and have a dragged-down, heavy feeling. Indifferent to loved ones. Chilly. Weepy. Dislike sympathy, prefer to be alone. Desires acidic things and chocolate. Better: vigorous exercise; eating; warmth; open air. Worse: during menstruation; missing a meal; pregnancy.

RHUS TOX

No. 1 Remedy for sprains and strains.
Stiffness, coupled with terrible restlessness. Pains usually around joints, which ache, feel sore, bruised. The pain gets worse on first movement, with a tearing or stitching sensation, but this eases after continued movement, provided it is not too strenuous. During colds, fevers or flu, a triangular red tip at the end of their tongue is an excellent confirmatory symptom. Children who need this remedy crave cold milk. Better: heat; gentle motion. Worse: damp, cold weather.

RUTA

No. 1 Remedy for injuries to tendons and bone surface. Ruta's action is deeper, but it has a less distinctive picture than Rhus Tox. It is less restless. Bone feels damaged. Useful for injuries to wrists; knees; ankles or bones with a thin covering of flesh (e.g shins). Better: for movement. Worse: lying on the affected part.

SILICA

No. 1 Remedy for forcing out splinters, etc.
In first aid treatment excellent for forcing foreign bodies out. In acute illnesses suits chilly types, who keep getting infections, which are very slow to clear up. Thirsty. Perspire easily. Better: heat. Worse: cold, damp, wet weather. If you have grommets or metal pins please consult a homœopath before taking this remedy.

STAPHISAGRIA

No. 1 Remedy following episiotomy.
Appear sweet and calm, but may feel angry, resentful, humiliated. Feel boundaries have been violated. Doesn't want to be touched. Very useful after cuts with a sharp instrument. Better: warmth; rest; breakfast. Worse: missing a meal; tobacco; exertion.

SULPHUR

Warm-blooded, wants doors and windows open. Empty sinking feeling in stomach at 11am. Desires sweets; spicy food. Burning pains. Offensive, corrosive, burning discharges. Itchy. Do not use routinely for skin complaints. In chronic skin complaints always see a qualified homœopath. Better: fresh air. Worse: warmth; bathing; 10-11am.

OTHER USEFUL PRODUCTS

Creams or Ointments:
Arnica - Can be used externally on **unbroken** skin. Reduces bruising and swelling.
Calendula - Use on cut, broken or sore skin. The "homœopath's antiseptic". A wonderful healing balm.
Urtica Urens - Very soothing on hot, itchy skin, caused by minor burns, sunburn or allergic reactions to insect bites and stings.

Bach Flower Remedies:
Rescue Remedy - A combination of five flower remedies, used to reassure and calm those who have had bad experiences or accidents. In many situations you can give this immediately, whilst you consider which remedy is most appropriate.

HOW TO FIND OUT MORE

If what you have read here interests you and you would like to prescribe for a wider range of complaints, you will need more detailed information. There are many excellent publications on Homœopathy, for example:

THE COMPLETE HOMŒOPATHY HANDBOOK
by Miranda Castro. (Macmillan ISBN 0-333-55581-3.)
Highly practical and authentic book.
Separate Repertory and 95 remedy Materia Medica.
HOMŒOPATHY, AN ILLUSTRATED GUIDE
by Ilana Dannheisser and Penny Edwards. (Element ISBN 1-86204-168-7). This practical, and clearly illustrated book is an invaluable guide to the effective use of the homœopathic remedies covered.

HOMŒOPATHY, MEDICINE OF THE NEW MAN
by George Vithoulkas
(Published by Thorsons ISBN 0722-509-898)
This is not a home-prescriber's manual, but its ideal for those who want more general, background information on Homœopathy.

It is also very worthwhile to learn basic First Aid techniques (for resuscitation, heart massage, to stop choking, etc). You may be able to attend classes locally. Alternatively,
THE FIRST AID MANUAL
(Dorling Kindersley ISBN 0863-189784) is a very comprehensive guide.

SEEING A QUALIFIED HOMŒOPATH

How do I find a qualified homœopath?
One way is to ask friends and neighbours if they have a local homœopath that they feel happy to recommend.
Otherwise contact either:

The Society of Homœopaths
11 Brookfield, Duncan Close
Moulton Park, Northampton NN3 6WL
Telephone: 0845 4506611
Fax: 0845 4506622
Enclose a large SAE and they will
send you their register.

The United Kingdom Homœopathic
Medical Association
Administration Office
6 Livingstone Road, Gravesend
Kent DA12 5DZ
Telephone & Fax: 01474 560336
They will send a register on request.

The Homœopathic Society
2 Powis Place
London WC1 3HT
They will send an information pack
about receiving homœopathic
treatment on the NHS and a list of
homœopathic doctors.

What happens during a consultation?

If you have a chronic, or frequently recurring complaint, the first consultation generally takes about one and a half hours. You begin by telling the homœopath what is troubling you. It is helpful if you can give as much detail as possible about your symptoms, including anything that makes them better or worse. If you have noticed any other changes in yourself (mood, anxieties, sleep, dreams, appetite, thirst, temperature) since the symptoms started; these can also be very useful. The homœopath will normally take a full medical case history from you and record details of any previous health problems in your family, going back to your grandparents. The aim of the consultation is to get an overview, not only of your complaint, but also of you as a person. Follow-up consultations usually last around forty-five minutes. They help you and your homœopath to assess your reaction to the previous remedy and decide how your treatment can best be continued. Sometimes, if the remedy is working well the homœopath may wait and not prescribe anything, but the information gathered during the appointment may well be used later on, in selecting the next remedy.

What happens after a consultation?

As stated earlier the key to successful prescribing is the Law of Similars. The symptom picture of the remedy is matched to the illness or injury and the closeness of the match determines the success of the cure. The first task is to carefully analyse the information collected in the consultation and select symptoms that are particularly characteristic or individual to your case. Once this is done, the homœopath uses two different kinds of reference books:

Repertories are books in which symptoms experienced by provers (testers) of homœopathically prepared substances are organised (both schematically and alphabetically). They have been expanding and improving steadily over the past two hundred years. So far over 1,000 different substances have been tested to see what symptoms they produce in a healthy person. A repertory provides a detailed index of symptoms to help narrow this huge number of substances down, by guiding the homœopath to those which best cover all the selected symptoms and traits. These particular substances can then be studied in depth in the *Materia Medica*. These are organised alphabetically, giving the names of each substance and describing them in great detail. This is where the final choice is made. Repertories and Materia Medica are now available on computer software which saves a lot of time when cross-referencing, but even so the search is likely to take quite a long time. For this reason the homœopath may not prescribe anything for you immediately, particularly if it is your first visit. If, however, your consultation was for an acute illness, the analysis will be simpler and the need for the remedy more urgent, so it will normally be prescribed there and then.

How many consultations will I need to have?

This is a very difficult question to answer and will depend on the individual case. However, one can generalise a little. Acute cases and injuries tend to respond very quickly once the correct remedy is found. The same is often true of more long-term problems which have a clear aetiology (ie. if you have never been well since a particular event). For chronic illness there is a rule of thumb that it may take up to one consultation for every year that you have had the complaint.

Should I stop taking all other medication?

It is important that you tell your homœopath about any medication that you are on. As a general rule, homœopaths do not advise you to stop taking prescribed drugs suddenly. Hopefully the need for these will lessen as treatment progresses and they can be gradually and carefully reduced. Since each case is different this is something that should be discussed during your consultations.

How can I tell if the homœopathic medicine is working or not?

Reactions to homœopathic medicines vary with the individual. Some experience a clear improvement in their symptoms very early on. Others find that their symptoms worsen for a time before improving (this is known as an aggravation). Still others find that their general sense of well-being increases, but the symptoms that they wanted cured stay the same. This is a very good sign as it shows the remedy is working at the most fundamental level and removing dis-ease. Eventually the original symptoms should disappear. Apart from general improvements (in sleep, digestion, mood etc.) homœopaths tend to look out for three particular things, which usually mean that there is a movement towards cure. The first is a shift in symptoms from above to below ie. from head to toe (eg. a rash moving down the body). The second is a shift from within out ie. from deeper parts of the body to the surface (eg. asthma changing to eczema). The third is that old symptoms start to reappear in reverse order. This is the equivalent of the body having a spring clean, clearing out old symptoms that have previously been suppressed. It will be a great help to your homœopath if you can mention any changes that you have noticed since taking the remedy. If you think you're likely to forget what has been going on, you could jot down a few notes throughout the month and bring them along to your next appointment.

Is it O.K. to self-prescribe when you are seeing a homœopath?

Self-prescribing can be very useful in treating acute illness or injury. Homœopaths treat the underlying weakness in the patient's constitution, this means that eventually you will have fewer acute illnesses. If you intend to see a homœopath regularly, please discuss self-prescribing with them before taking anything, as it may interfere with your treatment. Clearly, this does not apply in an emergency where the medicine can be taken immediately.